A Melanoma Patient's Survival Guide

Lemons
Really
Do
Make
Lemonade*

*You Just Have to Add a Little Sugar

by
Sally Welsh

©2004
Revised 2006

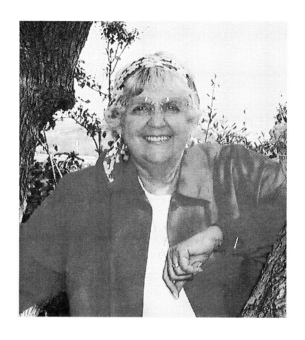

Sally Welsh lives with her husband, Terry, in Newport Beach, California. Her battle with melanoma has fostered in her an interest in helping others who are facing (or know someone who is facing) the ordeal of melanoma. She does not call herself an expert on the subject, nor a medical resource. She is, rather, just another "Traveler on the Road." She hopes her insight into the problem will help you and yours.

To contact Sally or to read more of her writings, please go to her website at: **www.themelanomaletter.com**.

My thanks to
the following who have
assisted me in the third printing of

Lemons Make Lemonade

Dolores and Bill Blurock
The Blurock Foundation

Janet Curci Walsh

and of course, my husband,
Terry Welsh

2006

Author's note:

Melanoma is being diagnosed in over 50,000 people a year in the United States alone. Melanoma will affect one in seventy-five people in California. That rate goes up each year. Melanoma can be a silent killer.

By sharing my experience, I hope to help you to make your melanoma journey a little easier. The suggestions I give are things I did which helped me to face this ordeal and improve my outlook on life.

My primary melanoma care was given by the **John Wayne Cancer Institute** in Santa Monica, California. I was in a vaccine clinical study there from 1999 to 2004.

Care for my general health has been done in my home town of Newport Beach, California, at **Hoag Memorial Hospital Presbyterian**. Physicians and Research Scientists at the Cancer Center at Hoag Hospital are also working on vaccine trials for melanoma.

As you read this book, I hope you will consider making a contribution to the melanoma research programs at either of these hospitals. This is an all out fight. I hope you will join me in the battle.

Sally Welsh

Contributions may be sent to:

John Wayne Cancer Institute	**Hoag Hospital Foundation**
Lemons Make Lemonade Fund	**Lemons Make Lemonade Fund**
2001 Santa Monica Blvd., Ste 860-W	**P. O. Box 6100**
Santa Monica, CA 90404	**Newport Beach, CA 92663**

Melanoma is rampant in our desert cities also. You can help to promote community education and awareness by a contribution to:

Eisenhower Lucy Curci Cancer Center
Patient and Family Support Fund "Lemonade"
3900 Bob Hope Drive
Rancho Mirage, CA 92270

FOREWORD

Into our lives, some rain must fall. We have heard that since childhood. Now that rain has fallen into my life, I have begun to reflect. Rain can be a tyrant, raging on its course, creating havoc, flooding and destroying all in its path. It can sweep away bridges, houses, people, and it can be relentless...or... it can feed and nourish, bring forth beauty, quench thirst, cleanse us and our surroundings, and grip our souls by its beauty. Sometimes it can do it all.

Melanoma is like that. It can rage and destroy, and it can create new beauty in your life.

In this book, I have tried to walk you through my journey into the dark clouds which brought rain into my life, and my gradual walk toward the rainbow. At times the relentless pounding seemed endless and just when I thought I would be swept away with the current, the clouds would part and the sun would come through. Sometimes it was only a brief respite from the rain, but it was always a reminder that the sun was just behind the clouds. As the clouds have come and gone, there have been moments of beautiful repose. Mother earth recovers from the onslaught, and so do we.

Your journey and mine are different, but our thoughts are probably similar. It is my hope that you will recognize yourself on some of my rainy days and that you will also join me in celebrating the sunlight that might not have been recognized in your pre melanoma days.

Drenched by rain, a seed will grow and eventually produce a lemon. By itself, the lemon tastes sour in your mouth. Lemons strongly flavor whatever they are near. Some lemons are used for garnish, purely decorative. Lemons are enjoyed as something with a tasty little tart flavor. For me, lemons are best when a little sugar is added. At that point, lemonade becomes a refresher, a cooler, a respite from the heat. It quenches thirst and renews.

It is your job and mine to take these lemons we have been handed, and to use them to flavor our lives At times we will encounter the bitter savor, but then we can add the sweet sugar that creates something which brings refreshment to our souls. By stirring the lemonade until the lemons lose their tartness, the sugar is not just sediment settled on the bottom of our glass. It is now pure enjoyment.

I'll pour, and you and I can raise a toast to our good health!

ACKNOWLEDGMENTS

This journey could not have been made without the continuing support of an army of people who have given me the chance for a future I might not have had, if I had been diagnosed with melanoma twenty five years ago. My thanks seem so inadequate, when I think of all the effort they have put into their work. Each one has a special place in my heart.

Anton J. Bilchik, M.D., Ph.D., F. A. C. S.
Assistant Director, Surgical Oncology, and Director of Gastrointestinal Research, at The John Wayne Cancer Institute. His knowledge and deft hands have saved my life more than once. He has been a gentle shepherd of my treatment.

Donald L. Morton, M.D.
Medical Director and Surgeon- in- Chief, The John Wayne Cancer Institute. His dreams and determination have saved the lives of countless cancer patients through his development of the Sentinel Node Procedure and the Melanoma Vaccine, both of which have benefited me.

Lynn Cambria, R.N.
Clinical Research Nurse at The John Wayne Cancer Institute. Her loving touch has eased my concerns and taken away the pain of my shots.

The Staff of The John Wayne Cancer Institute
From appointments, to lab tests, to hands on care, they are competent, professional, and caring.

The Family of John Wayne
Their dedication and effort to eradicate cancer is a remarkable tribute to their dad. Because of their enthusiasm, survival rates continue to rise. Their commitment is only excelled by their niceness.

Stan and Rae Cohen of Newport Beach
Friends who heard I was in trouble and were willing to go the extra mile

to help me map a direction for my treatment. They asked the questions, and I would not be at The John Wayne Cancer Institute without their research.

Edward G. Rohaly M.D.
Dermatologist in Newport Beach, California. Because of his willingness to take the extra time and do the proper procedures, my chances were improved immensely. He asked me if I had a book in me. Well, here it is.

The Staff of Dr. Rohaly's office
Their understanding and encouragement during difficult diagnostic times was a great support for me. I also thank them for getting test results to me as fast as possible.

The Staff of Hoag Memorial Hospital,
During my repeated visits for lab works and tests, they were helpful, always taking a friendly, personal interest in making my treatment easier.

The Vigilant Doctors and their Staffs, in Newport Beach, who have
used their medical specialties to watch over me. Every one of them has played a role in helping me to walk this road. I am so grateful for them and their care and interest in how they could help me to battle melanoma.

Gilbert Goodman, M.D., Internal Medicine
Gregory J. Katz, M.D., Internal Medicine
Sean S. Bahri, M.D., Ophthalmology
Kamal Batniji, M.D., F.A.C.S., Otorhinolaryngology
Donald R. Abrahms, M.D., Gastroenterology
Norman H. Bain, M.D., Gastroenterology
Jane Bening, M.D., Gynecology.
Weatherford B. Clayton, M.D., Gynecology
Dr. Richard Ardis, D.D.S.

Helene Bartosik, Jin Shin Acutouch Holistic Health Practitioner in Newport Beach

This country is great because people like you devote your lives to making a better life for others. Each one of you is a credit to your profession. You have my deepest thanks for helping me.

Thank you Lord, for blessing me with these caring individuals.

DEDICATION

This book is dedicated to
My Loved Ones
who make the fight worthwhile.

Terry

My husband and soul mate
whose
love and devotion is beyond measure

My Family

Chris

Doug and Mary

Charlie, Brittany, and Rebecca

who light up my life

TABLE OF CONTENTS

Author's Note
Foreward
Acknowledgments
Dedication

Lemons
Really
Do
Make
Lemonade*

*You Just Have to Add a Little Sugar

CHAPTER 1 - CLUB MELANOMA

So, you have joined an exclusive club you didn't want to join. Welcome!

There are a lot of members in this club. Every one of us has a story to tell. We know what it felt like to have a bomb dropped on us, and we can therefore empathize with what you are going through. We have walked the walk.

Though our stories are different, they follow a common thread. Most stories seem to follow the stages of grief. The patient starts with shock and ends with acceptance. The journey is full of potholes, but the experience isn't all bad. Beautiful things happen in the minds, hearts, and bodies of melanoma patients. Priorities change. Words that might never have been spoken are suddenly spoken. Faith grows. Beauty that was unseen is now seen. Life lived can become life lived Abundantly!!

One day, several months into my own melanoma treatment, I was sitting in the lab at the John Wayne Cancer Institute when a lady walked by. I will never forget the vacant, stunned look on her face. It was clearly a "Deer in the Headlights" look. She had joined the club. Suddenly I saw myself a few months before, and I realized that I had grown. I wanted to reach out to her and give her a hug. I had finished pledge class and was now a full member. It was time for me to help to make the road easier for others.

How could my journey become a tool to help? I am not a scholar, nor am I a medical professional. I do not have all the answers. What I do have, however, is a track record as a patient. My treatment is completed. I have had more experience with melanoma than many, six melanomas removed from my head and two surgeries for malignant lymph node removal.

If you are interested, the story of my club membership is told in Chapter 4 . It will be different from yours, but it will unite us because we are bonded together with our fears, our pain, our hopes. We know the secret handshake. We know the initiation rites. There is strength in using this bond to fight together and to reach out to one another. You are going to meet a lot of nice people in our club.

CHAPTER 2 - DEFINING THE MONSTER

Melanoma is the bad one when it comes to skin cancer. Most people know that. However, it amazes me how many people have little understanding of it. Most people think of melanoma as a dark black spot which begins to change. Well, melanomas come in many colors. They often have irregular edges, and when they evidence change, something is going on.

While melanomas can look like other skin cancers, they are really very different. Many skin cancers, like basal cells and melanomas, can grow laterally and down, but basal cell skin cancers do not enter the lymph system and travel to other parts of the body. They just spread wider and when finally removed, leave scars. They are a nuisance, and can be ornery, but they do not threaten your life. Melanoma does.

A tiny melanoma can begin to grow downward through your layers of skin, not stopping until it reaches your lymph system. Once it enters a lymph node, (or the blood) it is in contact with the rest of your body. If it decides to travel, it can destroy almost any organ it might hit. It can lie dormant, and just when it looks as if the coast is clear, "Bingo," it shows up on a chest x-ray, or a brain MRI. It can do this without its victim feeling a thing.

Most people believe that sun has a lot to do with melanoma, and in general, it can often be the culprit. A bad sunburn in your youth may come back to haunt you. Would you be surprised to know that melanomas can grow where the sun doesn't shine and can spread throughout the body undetected? There are women who have had primary melanomas in the vagina. Sometimes, the primary site of melanoma is never found.

A nice bald head is a sitting duck, but I have a full head of hair, and the scalp is where mine decided to surface. In all my years of wearing visors in the sun, it never occurred to me that the top of my head was so exposed. Actually, I have wondered if a severe chemical burn on my head from hair dye might have been a factor. I once frosted my own hair and when I took the "frosting " cap off all the newly frosted hair came with it. There was a bald spot the size of a pea right where my first melanoma grew. Hmmm...

Someone once remarked to me, "Oh, I have had melanoma, but it isn't cancer." I was astounded. Melanoma is cancer. It is the big "C." It is not something you nonchalantly say, "Oh, I'll just have my dermatologist remove it at my next checkup in six months." No. It is the one you have removed NOW. It is not something you ignore.

Another person showed me a spot where a melanoma had just been removed. When I questioned him about its depth, he really scoffed at me. He proudly showed me the healed wound. He said, "Look, it is all healed." He had no interest in the fact that the healing of the wound meant next to nothing. What went on below? How deep was it? Did he have tests to see if it had traveled? He didn't seem to grasp that the top layer was unimportant. His doctor might have told him, but it passed him right by.

Melanoma is also an area of medicine where we can help others. My husband wore bermudas to the dentist. The dentist glanced down at his leg and said, "You get to a dermatologist soon." It was a melanoma. Our dentist has found four of them. One night he saw a woman at a cocktail party and he couldn't take his eyes off her back. Luckily she was clad that night in a spaghetti strap summer dress. Embarrassed, he introduced himself to her and suggested she might want to see a skin doctor. The next week she called him to say thanks, because it was a melanoma. She did not even know the spot was there. She said, "You saved my life." She was probably right. We are our brothers' keepers.

You and I have our work to do. There is so much we can do to keep others out of our club. After all, it would be wonderful if our club remained small.

CHAPTER 3 - HELP, WHAT DO I DO?

If you have something suspicious on your skin, the first thing for you to do is to find a skin doctor, one who is most up to date in this rapidly changing battle. This skin doctor may be the individual who will save your life. This is a very important start on your melanoma journey.

Let's talk about doctors. They are wonderful. They are miracle workers. They are hard working. They care. They are overburdened. They have piles of medical journals to read at home at night. They can't possibly keep up with the written word and practice medicine too. We need to help our doctors to be current. A truly good doctor can learn from his patients too.

Many people have seen the same skin doctor for twenty or thirty years and speak of them burning off or scraping off things here and there. That is fine for most innocuous little spots. However, my melanomas never looked like melanomas. In fact, on one of them, my dermatologist even bet me his car that it would not be a melanoma. Unfortunately I won the bet. I told him I was a nice person, so I would let him keep his car. My melanomas had fooled him... more than once. Thankfully, he took the extra step on the side of caution. He did not just remove them as if they were nothing, he did punch biopsies to determine what they were before doing anything else. He was a good doctor. He did the right thing.

My case threw him challenges he hadn't had to face before. We are a team. He has studied hard to keep current and he has done a good job.

Let's reduce skin doctor shopping to three basic questions. Before the first visit to a dermatologist, the following would be important questions to ask:

> **"Will you be stripping me down and looking over my entire body, including my scalp?"**

> **"If you suspect I have a melanoma, will you be doing a punch biopsy?"**

> **"If my melanoma is level two or more in depth, will you be doing a Sentinel Node Procedure on me?"**

If any of those questions are met with a, "No," you might want to find a doctor who can say, "Yes," to them.

In the past, dermatologists only looked at the spots you showed them. Those days are gone. The doctor needs to take a look at all of your wrinkles, cellulite and barnacles.

The punch biopsy will give a much better reading of the very important depth of the melanoma, and the Sentinel Node Test may be able to pinpoint if and where it has spread. These are important questions, and perhaps your doctor may have missed this particular news in his reading. You need to know this before anyone cuts into you.

The other thing you have done by asking these questions is possibly save someone's life. If your doctor becomes interested in what you are telling him about this relatively new procedure, he will probably become involved in finding out what it is all about and educate himself. As I talk with melanoma patients all over the country, many have reported to me that they were the first to alert their doctors about the Sentinel Node procedure, and their doctors appreciated knowing about it.

When you do find that perfect doctor, you will have discussions about the best treatment and ultimately the choice will be made by you. You do need to know what is out there and to understand what has happened to you.

If the results of a punch biopsy return positive, you will make preparations to have the melanoma entirely removed, (hopefully accompanied by the Sentinel Node Test.) When the full pathology has been finished, you will then be presented with treatment options that range from doing nothing, to chemotherapy, and everything in between. The seriousness of your melanoma will determine your treatment in many cases, but in others, there will be several ideas for your treatment.

Soon you will be type cast as a Clark Level one through five and Cancer Stage I, II, III or IV. It all means something. It is important to know, but also important not to dwell on. There is a temptation to read statistics. Everyone wants to know what his chances are, but I have found that statistics are real mental setbacks. I remember one day when I began reading a chart about nutrition and melanoma. It was a happy, positive day. My eye reached the bottom of the chart and there were my statistics. There were those words and numbers telling me how long I might live. My happy day went from a sun shiny outlook to gloom in no time. This ushered me into a depression that went on for several days. I was at the point of cleaning out my closets.

Once we read our statistics we are caught up in them In my own case, I started ghoulishly to search on the internet for more figures, and I managed to get myself in a pretty doomsday state of mind. It would take me a long time to realize that, in my opinion, statistics are of no value to the patient. Oh sure, you might want to take another look at your will and get your papers in order...there is value to that. But...labeling yourself with death statistics will do you absolutely no good. I worked to get those images out of my mind and I don't go near them. I don't want to know them. It seems to me that they offer no positive input to our otherwise anxious minds.

When I finally came back to my own reality I said, "Hey, wait a minute. Those statistics include everybody. Those statistics don't give weight to the program I am on. Those people don't have the doctors I have. Those people don't have the prayer support I have. Those people may not be enrolled in yoga or biofeedback." I gradually pulled myself out of the slump. My advice, "Leave the statistics to the researchers." You do not need that negativity in your life. You will be far better off if you plan to be a Winner!

Make lemonade out of lemons. Share your story, just as I am sharing mine . People care. People want to know what to do if they should join this club. You can be an avenue to someone else's diagnosis. You may be the angel unaware, and you may be the catalyst to save someone else's life. Take it from me, there is no better feeling.

CHAPTER 4 - MY STORY

That little pink bubble on my scalp looked so innocent that I didn't even mention it to my skin doctor, Dr. Edward Rohaly. As usual during my yearly check-up, he had me strip myself, (yes, he takes a good look at the whole bod), gave me a thorough exam, (though not on my scalp), and pronounced me fine.

Your doctor should see all of you, in the buff. Melanomas are not always in the line of sight.

Returning home, I was annoyed that I had forgotten to show that tiny bubble to him. My inclination was to wait for my next checkup in six months. Something made me uneasy and pushed me to return the next week to have Dr. Rohaly check it out. I still wasn't concerned, and the "M" word was never mentioned. Wisely, he took a punch biopsy and sent me on my way. He had suspicions, but I didn't.

It should have concerned me when his nurse called to have me come in for the results, but I was preoccupied. Waiting that afternoon for Dr. Rohaly to appear, I reflected on the past few days. Just two days before, my mother had died after a five year bout with cancer. I had signed her cremation papers two hours earlier. It was a sobering chore and I was filled with pain. My husband and I had reflected about the fact that our care of her was over, she was at peace, and now we would have time for ourselves.

The door opened, and Dr. Rohaly came forward and kneeled before me. How strange. He looked up at me and said, "You have a malignant melanoma on your head." Of course I was there for the results of my biopsy, but I didn't even consider anything would be really wrong. That little pink bubble was resting on a beige pigmented base, a bad beige pigmented base. I just stared, wondering what this would mean. I had been going to cancer doctors for five years, watching my mother fight her battle. I knew cancer only too well. But that was her disease. I was much younger and ready to finally begin retirement with my husband.

Dr. Rohaly knew I was burdened by my mother's death and offered to drive me home. It was a kind gesture, but I needed to be alone to process this news. His attitude told me I was in serious trouble.

It was dark when I left his office and drove home wondering about my future. As I arrived home, something unusual happened. I walked in to find my two sons and my daughter-in-law chatting with my husband in the family room. They had just spontaneously dropped by as if God wanted me to be cushioned in that moment of grief upon grief. It was my first awareness that God had His hand on me. They accepted the news and comforted me.

Soon I would make my first mistake, while calling the office of my mother's oncologist. Foolishly, I asked the nurse if I should immediately see the oncologist, or if the melanoma should be taken out first. I had no business asking her that question and she should not have answered me. I never gave the oncologist the chance to counsel me. The nurse told me to have the melanoma taken out and to make an appointment to see the oncologist after that. That decision would surface to haunt me, because the oncologist might have suggested for me to have the Sentinel Node Test, a test we will explore later. I just plunged ahead arranging for the surgery with a local plastic surgeon.

My only thoughts were, "Get it out of there." Seeing the surgeon the next day, I arranged for surgery two days later, the day before my mother's services. The surgeon went on and on with the technicalities of my problem. He used terms not familiar to me. I remember just looking at him and saying to myself, "When is he going to tell me whether I am going to live or die?" Actually, it was hard to comprehend all he was saying. Had I been given the bottom line first, I might then have listened more carefully to the options. In fact, months later I told him that I didn't hear a thing he was saying because all I was interested in was whether I had a chance to live. He told me that he had mentioned the Sentinel Node Test, but because he wasn't then a believer in it, he didn't push it. It passed me right by. Six months later, he was a believer.

Because I did not process his words, my mistakes multiplied. I did not read about melanoma. I did not research any treatment. I did nothing but prepare my final goodbye to my mother.

The surgery, centrally located on my scalp, about an inch into my hairline above my forehead, was rather scarring. In fact, my husband did not let me look at it for quite awhile. It was a divot larger than a silver dollar, sunken in, and covered by a skin graft taken from my upper leg. It would be a permanent bald spot. It was ugly. But at least I could rest in the news that, "My margins were clear," or so we thought.

Never being one to fuss with my hair, there was a new challenge. My style is "Wash and Wear" haircuts. All of a sudden there was this thing to cover up. Thank goodness for scarves, Learning to fold them and use them as wide enough headbands to cover my problem was not natural for me. It felt as if others might think I was trying to court a new image, to be someone I was not.

Attending my mother's services the day after my surgery, with a scarf tied over my rather large wound, I felt self conscious. The pastor made a short announcement of my problem, but then asked attendees to devote the day to my mother and not to my problem. I tried to do the same.

It came time for my first visit with the oncologist. Upon entering his waiting room, I was suddenly overcome with:

Today I am one of THEM!!!

How did this happen?

There has been a mixup.

I was the strong one who had brought my mother to this oncologist's office for five years.

I was the jaunty one.

I had all my hair.

I had energy.

I made her appointments, asked the questions for her, felt her frail hand take my arm to steady her.

I drove the car.

I picked up the prescriptions.

I dragged home all those cans of Ensure.

Whoa! This was not part of the bargain.

I have walked this road before, in the company of another. I don't need to walk it again.

But, it is me.

I am the patient.

That is my chart.

When is it time for my vacation?

When I was finally ushered into the oncologist's office, he gently explained my case to me, telling me that he thought the best plan for me was to be put me on a year of interferon, giving myself daily shots. It would have side effects, causing me to have a year of feeling as if I had the flu. Blindly, I agreed. It would begin when my surgery had healed.

About four weeks later I was talking about theater tickets with my friend Rae Cohen. We shared what was going on in our lives. Five minutes after we hung up, her husband, Stan Cohen, was on the phone. "Sally, tell me about it. What are your numbers? How deep is it? Give me the details, I want to call our physician son, (Gordon Cohen, a pediatric heart transplant surgeon), in London."

That Sunday night I arrived home to a message from Stan, "Call me whenever you get in. You have an appointment with our son's best friend from medical school. He is a Surgical Oncologist at the John Wayne Cancer Institute at St. John's Hospital in Santa Monica, California. I have been discussing your case with him today. Your appointment is on Tuesday!"

It was only an hour and a half away from me. I would be there!!!

I would learn that the John Wayne Cancer Institute is the largest melanoma treatment center in the United States and that they have treated more patients than anyplace else in the country. They had been working for years on a vaccine to help the patient's system to build up an immunity to melanoma. It was still in the protocol (experimental) stage, but they were seeing some great success.

People from all over the world were coming to them for this exciting treatment. (See page 77 for vaccine update.) Over time I would encounter them as they arrived from Africa, Holland, South America, Greece and all over the United States.

It was important for me to see these professionals before starting any other treatment, because another treatment might make me ineligible for their vaccine. I would not be starting the interferon.

On Tuesday, Dr. Anton Bilchik walked into my life, and took me on as a patient. I knew I was in the right hands. This kindly act on the part of my friend Stan had opened the door for me to be treated by an incredible team of doctors, nurses, receptionists, lab technicians, and medical personnel who would work like an army charging into battle. I felt surrounded by capable, encouraging hands. I began the long process of letting go of fear and letting the experts get to work.

Where had the fear come from? Why was I so eager to wallow in a cloud of doom. It didn't take me long to realize that part of it was that I let myself be drawn into that well of statistics for my survival.

Because of the depth of my melanoma, I was considered a Clark level three. There are five depth levels to the Clark scale and level three moves into a level of real concern. About the only thing that was good news was that it was not a level four or five. I was labeled

Stage two Cancer (out of four stages), because my melanoma had not spread to my lymph nodes.

Dr. Donald Morton had been working on a melanoma vaccine since the early sixties. One day a distraught mother arrived, having had a serious melanoma on her arm, with sixteen positive lymph nodes. She had been given six months to live. She would not see her sons raised. She had no hope. Dr. Morton told Peggy Maddox that his vaccine was ready for trial and asked if she would like to be the first. She is here today, an active woman I often see at John Wayne Cancer Institute functions. She is living hope for melanoma patients.

The vaccine has been created from the cells of many melanoma patients. Peggy's first dose of the vaccine was twenty five million cells of live melanoma which had been radiated so that it couldn't reproduce. Over the years, more clinical trials have been used throughout the world to get that number down. My program consisted of being injected with one million cells of the live, radiated melanoma, monthly. Though the shots sting somewhat like bee stings, the pain disappears within minutes. They are administered in the lymph areas under the arms and on both sides of the groin...eight shots. I have not experienced any side effects like chemotherapy patients have.

Things were going great as my seventh series of shots approached. I was filled with pleasant anticipation. Some patients were considered finished at that point and I was sure that I was doing so well that I would be one of those lucky ones.

My worries were nearly behind me.

It was time for my regular three month check with my

dermatologist, Dr. Rohaly, and I had no worries there either. I did, however, feel a slight rough spot on my scalp, near the old site. I waited as Dr. Rohaly ran his hands through my hair and in retrospect I wish I had waited just a few minutes longer to see if he would find it. I raised my hand and said, "What about this?" He began to examine this rough spot with greater interest and thought it was something benign. Because of its placement, he did think a punch biopsy was in order. I was calmed by his description that it looked like something innocuous. Well, it wasn't. It was a new melanoma, totally unrelated to the first one.

It unnerved me a little to realize that I had found both of my melanomas myself. Then my oncologist told me that ninety percent of melanomas are found by the individuals themselves. It is important that we know our own bodies.

Dr. Bilchik and Dr. Rohaly spoke and surgery was scheduled. This time I would have the Sentinel Node procedure first. Emotionally the thought of going through surgery all over again hit hard. I had mentally prepared that it was time to see my plastic surgeon about reconstructive surgery on the first site, and now I was headed for another invasive procedure.

CHAPTER 5 - THE SENTINEL NODE

We need to take a moment to explore the Sentinel Node Procedure. It is imperative you understand it before my story continues.

This incredible Sentinel Node test, again a product from Dr. Morton's research, has shown such promise. It can make the difference between life and death. In my own less than medical terminology, I will try to explain it to you. Hopefully, you know all about it by now from your own research.

You have just discovered something strange on your body. Perhaps it has changed color or size. Something is calling you to have it checked out. First step is to the dermatologist. Some of this is a repeat from the first chapter, but I hope to make you very clear on what important information it is for you to know. The Sentinel Node test has been around for a long time, and there are still dermatologists who have no knowledge of it. I am a lay person. I am not a medical person. I can help you to ask some questions and start you on a path, but I emphasize that my only purpose is to get you to ask the right questions before anyone cuts into you. You need to know your options before you start.

This is the reason why the three questions, (previously suggested in Chapter 3), for you to ask your doctor, are supremely important. First, since depth is critical for a melanoma, a punch biopsy will do a better job of determining depth than just scraping some of it off. The punch is simply a pencil like device. The area is anesthetized and this device pulls out a plug, much like a cork out of a wine bottle. From that core tissue, depth can be determined. A level one melanoma the size of a nickel can be much less lethal than a pinhead sized one that is deep into level five. You need to know depth.

Basically, the Sentinel Node test is done most successfully before the entire melanoma is removed. The patient is taken to radiation where the area is deadened and then radiated. The doctor uses his fingers to stimulate the area to cause the lymph nodes to begin to show up on a screen. They look like raisins. The radiologist selects the lymph nodes where he feels the melanoma would travel. It is just like a railroad train headed for the round house.

The patient is taken to surgery for removal of the melanoma, but before the melanoma is removed, blue dye is injected into it. The doctor watches the train of blue dye follow a track down to one of these "raisin" nodes. The node the train selects is then designated the Sentinel Node. From that node, evil cells may begin to travel out of the round house on their special tracks, ready to target something else in the body. That is where trouble begins, because those evil cells want to reach your liver, your lungs, your brain... something really important.

If the Sentinel Node shows the presence of any malignant cells, another surgery will be performed to remove nodes around the Sentinel Node to see if any other nodes have been affected. If the Sentinel Node is clear, the conclusion is that the malignant cells did not travel beyond that node, and the cancer can then be deemed gone. No further surgery is necessary.

There is more good news. Because of the efforts of Dr. Armando Giuliano at the John Wayne Cancer Institute, the Sentinel Node test is now being routinely used in the field of breast cancer. Since 1996, hundreds of thousands of breast cancer victims have had their lives saved by this test. Spread the word!!

Keep an ear open for the next news from Dr. Bilchik. He is working on a protocol program to foster use of the Sentinel Node Test to track any spread of colon cancer. We should all pray for his success on this project.

With Dr. Bilchik in charge, surgery on the second melanoma on my head would include the Sentinel Node procedure, which I had not had before my first melanoma was removed.

As I was taken through the Sentinel Node procedure, I was grateful for the modern technology that provided such fine care for me. The radiologist created a profile of me on a screen and then injected something radioactive into the melanoma. It created a burst of black on the screen. He then pummeled behind and in front of my right ear, encouraging the radioactivity to spread. Soon several raisin looking spots (the lymph nodes) developed on the screen both in front and in back of my ear. He selected two or three spots behind my ear and put little tape markers on them. This was apparently where he expected the blue dye to go when injected.

I returned upstairs to await surgery. During surgery I was under general anesthesia while the blue dye was then injected and observed as it drained to three lymph nodes behind my ear. A frozen section indicated that the nodes were clear, but they were removed and further testing was done . They were confirmed all clear.

The Stage I, 0.8 mm deep melanoma was then removed, and a skin graft about the size of a quarter was taken from my neck.

Returning home that night, I felt relieved to have this behind me, I was on vicodin and an antibiotic. Thursday night I went sailing. Friday night my husband and I dined out with friends. All was well.

We went to bed about eleven and the nightmares began. I was up eight times during the night, having been terribly upset by dreadful scenes. I just couldn't seem to get over them. They ranged from self-destructive behavior to disasters and being victimized by horrible crime. Since my dreams are primarily happy, this was frightening to me. In the morning I didn't want my husband to even go to the market. I was afraid, dissolving in tears easily. At 10:30 A.M. Dr. Bilchik called to check on my status and I was able to tell him that I was having a meltdown. I have no idea what an LSD trip might feel like, but my imagination told me that it must feel like what I was experiencing. Dr. Bilchik suggested abandoning the vicodin and antibiotic, and using a tame tranquilizer to get myself back to normal. As the day wore on things continued to improve. I wouldn't call myself stable, but at least moving forward. Apparently vicodin is not the drug for me.

About a week later bouts of diarrhea and terrific stomach cramps arrived. The cause... facing a mammogram which I dreaded because they were watching something abnormal which had occurred just before my first melanoma. I was very frightened they would find something, and resorted to being was very tearful. I just didn't think I could handle another blow. To my great joy, it was just fine and the relaxation could begin..

Seeing my internist during this period, I dealt with all sorts of symptoms such as stomach cramps, dizziness, heart type anxiety. It is hard to differentiate between my vertigo, panic disorder , esophageal reflux and things that could possibly be heart related. My blood pressure had risen to about 169/80 at the Cancer Institute since starting on the vaccine, but thankfully it was close to normal in my internist's office. I did not appear to be handling my life very well.

The second surgery had taken its toll on me emotionally and I tried to reason why. My analysis is that I believe that this entire

22

drama falls in the category of grief. I had buried my grief. I really did not have time to grieve for my mother when my own body was invaded. I just marched from her disease to mine. My mother was ready to give up her fight and I was at peace with her passing. I had not grieved her loss. I hadn't grieved over my melanoma. A health problem is reason for grief. It should be grieved.

Throughout those days I tried never to say or have an attitude of, "Why me?" I always said, "Why not me?" People would say how great I was handling it, but inside I felt very fragile.

Writing a letter to alert others about melanoma was a form of therapy for me. It gave me a proactive way to work out my emotions. Busying myself at my desk, I talked to anyone who would listen to me. I really tried to be positive. I'd like to think I did a good job.

In reality, I was avoiding, burying, ignoring, my deep feelings. Can you relate to that? Could I really be angry? Hmmm...that's a thought.

While sailing along toward health several months after my second surgery, my world was jarred once again. On the outer rim of my "silver dollar scar," Dr. Rohaly noted a new bump had arisen. A punch biopsy revealed that my margins had not been clear. Tiny micro cells had begun to bloom. The news was good and bad. Bad, of course! Who wants another melanoma? On the other hand, Dr. Bilchik felt that this might be a blessing in disguise, as he would do a Sentinel Node test on the assumption that the new "in transit" would be on the same tree trunk as my original melanoma. The test originally denied to me would be done, thank goodness. My excitement was short lived. Soon I would find out I had big troubles.

This second melanoma on my original site enabled Dr. Bilchik to use the Sentinel Node test to track the melanoma to a lymph node behind my left ear. The frozen section deemed it clear, but high powered microscopes in the later pathology found a micro-metastasis. It was contaminated. He removed that node and eventually twenty-eight other nodes down my neck, to make sure the contaminated node had not moved on to others. Thankfully only the one node was affected, but it was a Time Bomb we would never have found without the Sentinel Node being identified. Since the lymph node was infected, I had now moved from Stage Two cancer, to Stage Three.

Over the next few months three more "in transits" arrived on the edge of my "clear margin." Because the node test had been done, Dr. Bilchik did not feel it necessary to repeat it. My depths were now at Level Four (out of Five).

During the period of 18 months, I had eight surgeries. Then I began about two years of uneventful routine. I reached my graduation day from the vaccine, It was a glorious day. I would leave in two days for a month in Hawaii. No more vaccine.

Dr. Bilchik gave me my graduation speech. It was wonderful. He turned to walk from the room to arrange for my last vaccine, He had his back to me when again, something turned him around. He walked back to me to take one last check of my lymph nodes in my neck. His finger immediately landed on a hard spot and his face fell. He got the pathologist for needle biopsies, but there was no evidence of melanoma. He said, "I can't let you go to Hawaii. I think that node is melanoma and we must take it out." Two days later I had it out and it was melanoma. One lethal node in a pocket of nine. Eight nodes were clear. God had tapped Dr. Bilchik on the shoulder as he started to leave that room. I am sure of it.

Decision time. Was the vaccine not working on me, or did the vaccine hold the one node from going on to the others? We choose to think that this was an "in transit" that got away and tried to establish its own Sentinel Node. We choose to think the vaccine is working. Only God knows, but I am back in the vaccine program and happy to be there.

Every three months I see Dr. Rohaly for an all over check, with much time spent on the scalp, as well as the rest of my body. He is very careful to keep an eye on me.

My ophthalmologist, Dr. Sean Bahri, also watches intently over my eyes every four months, because my melanomas were on my head, near my eyes.

I see Dr. Bilchik every three months, and my Nurse, Lynn Cambria does monthly checks on my lymph nodes. Certain blood tests are also done on a regular basis, along with chest x-rays.

My regular doctors and my dentist, also watch over me vigilantly. They know the consequences of unattended melanoma, and maintain a careful eye. It is my responsibility to mention my concerns to them.

So there you have it, one person's melanoma journey. Your journey will be different than mine, but the process and the emotions will no doubt be very similar. I hope you only have one melanoma to deal with.

I don't think much about my future. I think about today. If my mind drifts to ominous thoughts, I quickly return to today. Today is great, and I don't want to miss a moment of it. Don't you miss anything either.

CHAPTER 7 - ARE YOU ANGRY?

Time has taught me that one must go through all the steps of grief, and ANGER was one I had skipped. Getting the second melanoma finally made me angry. I felt like I was a good sport and was doing everything to show God I had accepted my fate. Right when I was almost at the finish line there was another blow. That really didn't seem fair. But I buried it and where did it surface? Bad dreams. Stomach cramps. All sorts of ills. My body rebelled when my conscious mind didn't know how to express this anger.

Once recognized, I began to read about anger. An enemy is so much easier to deal with when it is identified. I searched for articles and books dealing with anger. The "hit a pillow" stage was one suggestion that had intrigue. Instead, I decided to journal. Journaling has helped me to sort it all out. It felt so good to spill it all out on paper.

I am ANGRY.

I want to feel good again.

This is MY time with MY husband, and it wasn't supposed to be spent in doctors' waiting rooms.

I don't enjoy martyrdom. I don't know if people like to be around people who are "damaged." It might be catching.

I just want to be me.

I don't like to worry, but it is always there lurking, wanting to get the best of me.

I have been told that my hats and scarves flatter me. But I know why they are there. They are almost a pronouncement, like a scarlet letter.

Hats and scarves are sometimes binding and uncomfortable.

I didn't get to go on a vacation cruise in the San Juans.

Our Hawaii trip had to be shortened because of my treatment.

My body is scarred.

My hair is ugly.

I don't go to fun things anymore. I go to doctors. I sit in waiting rooms.

My shots sting like eight bee stings each time I go for a treatment.

It is a long drive in traffic for my vaccine shots.

I don't like to have to be so dependent on my husband.

I love being loved. I hate being pitied.

I want to feel good enough to entertain again.

I want to have energy to keep up with my grandchildren.

I am becoming a one-issue bore.

Maybe if I get this put on paper, it will begin to take its rightful place, in the deep recesses of my mind.

I am angry, but I am not going to stay angry.

I acknowledge that this was a raw deal... for me... for anybody who has to go through it.

I am ready to fight back.

The Twenty Third Psalm says, "Thou preparest a table before me in the presence of mine enemies." Mine enemies are those dumb melanoma cells and you know what? That table, that feast, was prepared for me, not them. I intend to sit at that table that has been prepared for me and stare down those hungry cells. They simply do not get to participate in my feast. They can just starve to death!

This is the time "Thou makest me to lie down in green pastures."

This is the time, "Thou restoreth my soul."

This is the time, "My cup runneth over."

When I put away my anger, "I shall dwell in the house of the Lord, forever."

Once again I grasp life. I was healed in spirit. I had another ugly scar on my head, but I could handle that.

You've been diagnosed! That benign report you had hoped for stated, "Malignant Melanoma." It doesn't take long for the Mind Games to begin

Initially, it's hard to believe. You don't feel any different than you did when you walked into the doctor's office. Yet, your life has changed. They're going to take the melanoma out of there. Small scar. "No big deal." And for some of you that will be true. But then there are the rest of us.

I remember walking around that first week obsessed with, "How long do I have?" I finally started to take one day at a time. Upon awakening, I would think. "I don't think I am going to die today." Gradually I would say to myself, "I think I can make it for another week." Pretty soon a month had passed and I speculated in awe, "Maybe I can make it another month."

It sounds silly to me now, but that is the first step I took. "Maybe I can!" Now it is your turn. "Maybe you can!"

I started to research on the internet and found out that I was learning more than I wanted to know. There is a line in there somewhere that the patient does not need to cross until he is ready. We want to know enough to be knowledgeable, but not enough to make ourselves more scared than we already are. My way of handling it was that the doctors could be the scientific ones, not me.

My own case was such a roller coaster that my mind became my worst enemy. Time after time I was told that everything was okay, only to learn ten days later that there was a new problem. Between the statistics, (which worsened after each of my eight surgeries), and being given the impression that things were okay when they were not, I had a hard time controlling my outlook. Simply put, I was afraid to be positive.

"Your margins are clear." I didn't think another thing about it. But you know, they can't test every single little cell. My margins weren't totally clear. "Your lymph nodes are clear." Oops, they weren't. In fairness to the doctors I will say that not everything can be found in the operating room by just frozen tissue.

Thank God they pursued further testing of my tissue with special high powered microscopes or they would never have found these remnants.

It became apparent I needed to go to work on my mind. The stress was eating me up. Hardest to bear was the waiting. On a regular basis there was a chest x-ray, cat scans, brain MRI's, all sorts of tests and I was almost incapacitated waiting for the results of them. I would not allow myself to even hope they would be clear. I had tried that too many times. People were always asking, "How are you doing?" Truthfully, I did not know. It seemed as if every time I said "Great," the bomb would fall.

One vaccine treatment day a relief nurse was giving me my vaccine and said to me, "So what stress were you under to bring this upon yourself?" The mind had been a participant in my problem and it needed to be treated too.

A friend referred me to a professional in biofeedback. It was a place where I could let my hair down. A kindly psychologist listened to my fear and validated that I wasn't crazy to be acting the way I was. He acknowledged that I truly had been on a roller coaster. As he worked with his equipment and I could see my brain waves on the screen, I, too, could see the devastation my mind was causing me. It didn't matter that my concerns were valid. What did matter was that I needed to begin to control my reactions to this fear.

It was revealing to see how different the conscious mind was from the subconscious or unconscious mind. I was taught how to focus to lower my stress level, and to use certain exercises of the mind to do it.

He taught me at one point to visualize a spinning gyroscope honing out the malignancy and to feel it whirring around the edges of it and getting rid of every last contaminated cell. He had me concentrate on literally sanding away the cancer until it was totally gone. It may sound funny, but it worked. It gave me a sense of power that I was getting all of it out of there.

Somewhere along the way there was an attempt to work on my nutrition, though I still do not have a handle on that. Sugar feeds cancer and it is so important for a cancer patient to get rid of that obsession, but I find it very hard. There is something psychological about pampering myself with a sweet. It is a feel good treat for me. Too many good intentions. Too little commitment. This will be a continuing challenge for me while walking my journey. Good luck to you.

An easy yoga class was the next step and I could feel the good it was doing.

Involuntarily I would hear my mind saying, "This is so good for me." I learned to deeply relax and meditate, concentrating on my own faith.

I have come to love the melding of Eastern and Western medicine.

This in no way undermines my confidence in my doctors, because of the concrete information they have from my tests and scans. There is room to believe that the East has reached the untouchable realms of our energy fields, and can help us.

While I was caring for my mother, a good friend led me to acutouch to help me to keep myself healthy. Acutouch is a form of acupressure which requires no disrobing. The belief is that energy meridians run throughout our bodies. As long as the energy flows freely from A to B, we are well. When energy is blocked , we do not feel as well. By listening to energy pulses, a true professional can determine what area of the body is not functioning well.

I always felt uplifted when I attended a session. Perhaps if I had done it earlier, my system would have been built up enough to fight off the melanoma on its own. Apparently it is well known that we all have cancer come and go in our lives, but most of the time, our immune systems are strong enough to fend it off. It is when we let ourselves down or don't take care of ourselves that we become vulnerable.

Let me give you an example of acutouch. Probably two years after my mother died, I awakened one morning sobbing over the loss of her. I didn't know where it came from. She hadn't been on my mind the day or night before. I had my tears for about a half hour and proceeded to go about my day. I arrived mid afternoon for my acutouch session. I said nothing of my morning tears and by then I had been on my daily errands, and there was no evidence of my episode. My pulses were read, and I was told that we would work on the heart meridian that day. Alarmed, I asked what was wrong with the heart. I was told, "The heart is the center of grief, and I think you are dealing with grief today." I couldn't believe my ears. She had no way of knowing what I had gone through in the morning. I went from just a believer to a very strong believer, and I have continued to go to her for wellness.

Would you like my sure cure for getting to sleep? There are many ways to "Count Sheep." Promise me you won't laugh at my way. Since I have spent many hours looking at the ceiling, and problems always seem so much worse at night, I have devised a scheme that is not only fun, but lulls me off to sleep. My scheme has allowed me to run through my life a second time. People who have not had their health threatened have no need to do that. I, however, think I am getting a two for one sale, and there are lots of things in my life I am enjoying for a second time.

I started very simply. I decided to relive every trip I have ever taken.

Example:
Our first trip in our new Ford camper van was up the Oregon Coast. Our boys were three and five and most of the trip they wore their prize leather lederhosen short pants. They hardly required cleaning. We just shook the dirt out and stood them up in the corner. At that age the boys could stand and walk around inside the van. We would pull into a campsite, usually in the tall trees, and begin the process of outdoor cooking. Daytime was spent roaming the driftwood covered beaches looking for agates, shells and of course odd shapes of driftwood. We watched sea lions and seals.

We ate chowder at Moe's and visited the ancient aquarium in Newport. Watching the ships come through the raging waters into the calm seas of Depot Bay was scary and fascinating. Of course we had to stock up on the town specialty, salt-water taffy.

Those are 35 year old memories and I can relive them as if they were yesterday.

I have been on all my European trips a second time, to mountain cabins, Hawaii, Canada, Tahiti—you name it—all in the most minute detail.

I have tried to remember every teacher I had in school and what each classroom looked like. I visualized the puppet show we gave in fifth grade, what we did at recess, riding my bike home on a snowy day my second grade year when the school caught on fire, the carnival in our back yard, high school parties and football games. I have lived these experiences twice, and I have had a wonderful time doing it.

How many friends of your youth can you remember? What did your homes look like when you were growing up? How were they decorated? What is the oldest article of clothing you can remember? How many types of big cats can you visualize? God was a creative genius to engineer spiders making webs, or perhaps eels. How does the cobra move that big body around? Giraffes and kangaroos are fun to think about.

My most recent venture took me into rocks. I started with the Rockies and Mount Rushmore, and went all the way to Michaelangelo's David in Florence. Rocks bring us such beauty, but they work for us, and dikes, foundations and roads are built from them. I worked my way all the way to sand. It took me many nights to explore rocks and then I began adding water to the sand. Soon I was off on the importance of water to us.

If you try this, you will see that the list will grow as long as your imagination does. It is like a personal tour of our world, and others aren't taking time to really examine it, just for fun. When I feel myself drifting into negative thoughts I quickly go to a new subject I can really get lost in.

For my moments of very deep concern, I always turn to prayer, pouring out my concerns to the Father. I know He is listening.

Did I lose you on these last paragraphs? Before you write me off, try one of my ideas and see if you don't sleep like a babe.

An absolute must in any patient's agenda is the reading of "Love, Medicine, and Miracles," by Dr. Bernie Siegel. During a particularly low period, I had been told to get that book. I didn't do it. When we arrived at the home where we have vacationed in Hawaii for fifteen years, I felt myself drawn to their bookcase. I had always ignored it, There, at eye level was Dr. Siegel's book. I laughed out loud and said, "Well God, I guess you really wanted to have me read this book." I did, and it took my outlook from despair to joy. I can't say enough about it.

My husband and I were in the habit of watching the eleven o'clock news. I would try to go to sleep with the weight of the world on my shoulders. It was all war and murders, and violence. What a thing to dwell on just prior to sleep. No wonder I was having a hard time. Turn it off!!!

TV sitcom reruns are available at eleven P.M. We began to laugh our way to sleep. Norman Cousins brought about his own cure through laughter, and he really had a good idea. The nights have become much more a time for laughter.

Come to think of it, the morning paper isn't too cheerful either. I began to just give it a glance. I didn't want to be regarded as a total dummy. A glance is enough in most cases. No one needs to know the sordid details of murders, rapes, shootings. Life is a better place without the morning news.

I was on a roll. No more gloomy message movies with tragedy upon tragedy. No more violent shoot'em ups. I will take a "Sleepless in Seattle." any day, exiting the theater with a smile on my face.

Continuing to deal with inquiries about my health, I began saying, "Today is great!!" The more I said it the more I realized that, "Today really is great." We don't need to think beyond that.

Today was great for all the people who went into those towers. They did not get up that morning with a sense of doom, though they were just hours from death. The astronauts aboard Columbia were full of exhilaration on February 1, 2003. My own father, and interesting enough my daughter-in-law's father, both died on the first tee of the golf course, having a whale of a time. We should all concentrate on the moment. I began to lie in bed at night and force myself to think of something wonderful that had happened that day. I went over the day with a fine tooth comb. There was always something to celebrate about the day. Why hadn't I done that before?

Another thing that I have trained myself to do is to walk the horizon. During my first months it seemed as if I lived in great hope, then was plunged to despair, then elevated to hope. It was very hard on me emotionally. It was always mountain peaks and valleys. The swings were really affecting me. I began to concentrate on not going too high if I had had good news, and conversely not going so deep when the news was bad. Sometimes I felt guilty celebrating a victory with only modest enthusiasm, but it really worked for me to try to keep my emotions closer to the center line.

I still live my life that way. It's a great way to live!! I hope you can live that way too.

CHAPTER 9 - MY FAITH

As I have walked my walk, I have become more comfortable with life and death. I have been asked how my faith has helped me to cope with this continuing battle. My faith is what carries me through the rough times. It soothes me during fitful times. When I ask for the peace that passes understanding, somehow a calmness comes over me.

I cannot fathom what it must be like to face a life threatening disease without faith in God. As a Christian, my faith is based on the teachings of Jesus Christ. I cling to His eternal promises.

For those of you of other faiths, I reach out my hand to you. I happen to be a Presbyterian married to a Roman Catholic. Throughout our married life we have followed some advice I read long ago. We celebrate and enjoy that which we have in common, and respect and include one another in those areas where our beliefs are different. It has worked for us.

September 11, 2001 joined all of our hands together as we sought to find common ground against an enemy. As you and I face our health issues we know that patients, doctors and medical personnel of all faiths are joined together to battle the same evil. Whatever the faith, the goals are the same. We need to pray for each other and for those who are trying to save our lives.

Great comfort has come to me from the scriptures. Somewhere along the way I came upon a biblical promise that has meant much to me. It was God's gift to me. It has been on my desk since the day I first read it.

1 Peter 5:8-11

And the God of all grace

Who called you to His eternal glory in Christ,

After you have suffered a little while, will Himself restore you

And make you strong, firm and steadfast.

To Him be the power forever and ever.

Amen

Reading it filled me with instant courage. I might have to suffer, but I had the promise of restoration. Possibly that restoration might not be of this world, but I will be restored. My outlook changed.

My husband and I read the One Year Bible cover to cover, and I began to see myself as a speck on the time line of the history of mankind. For me, it confirmed that what is really important is to concentrate on living each day I am given on that time line and to live it in tune with God. By truly living each day, I began to climb back up the mountain.

I asked God to keep me close and to help me to do His will as I followed this journey. I asked Him to help me to accept whatever is in my future.

In the morning, before arising, I go deep into prayer. I take time at first to analyze some great thing God has created for His people, something beautiful. I picture it and take it in. I visualize and appreciate its presence in my world. I thank God for creating it to be enjoyed...the sea, a country scene, sunrises or sunsets. Don't you think that God would like to know we notice and appreciate His creation, before we bombard Him with requests?

I pray for my family, my friends, those in painful situations, in grief, in poverty, in war zones, at bedsides, in pain. I pray for our leaders making such monumental decisions, so much on their shoulders. I pray for those who lay their lives on the line to protect us. I pray for doctors and scientists and health care professionals... mere humans, from whom we expect godly miracles.

All of our problems diminish when we think of others.

My prayers always include all my soul mates with melanoma. The list continues to grow in an alarming way. I specifically pray for my own doctors, nurses, and the scientists who work for the cure or containment of melanoma.

Lastly, I pray for myself, always "Thy will be done." I want to accept this cross, to carry it with dignity, to be the servant God wants me to be. I do add a prayer, asking Him to make me well. After all, He wants us to pray specifically. Mostly I ask Him for the courage to face anything He has for me and to walk through it with me, that I might honor Him.

Do you know who Simon of Cyrene was? He was a simple soul who happened to be standing beside the road as Jesus carried His cross to Calvary. A Roman soldier pulled him out of the crowd to help Jesus to carry the cross. Simon could have said, "Why me?" He could have run. He chose to accept it as an honor to carry the heavy cross of the Lord. I would like to visualize myself accepting the melanoma like Simon accepted the cross. I would like to think that my acceptance of this cross would please the Lord. I pray to

41

be as willing as Simon.

There is a prayer ministry in our church. When I pick up the prayer list and see that people are praying for me, it touches me deeply. What a gift to know that others care enough to pray for us. So many studies are going on now as to whether prayer really does work for healing. Thus far, even skeptics are beginning to believe in the power of prayer.

I carefully go over the names on the prayer list, praying for their needs.

My faith is not an accident. My parents were people of great faith. I was led to the church by them each Sunday. I was raised to believe. Their faith was real. It was lived in our home and in the community. My parents had their priorities in order. My parents could be counted on to practice their faith. They were not just religious on Sunday. They walked their faith in the way they treated others.

My father always took an active role in the life of the church. My mother took her role as a care giver for those in need.

My mother suffered most of the five years of her cancer, but she was not one to complain She was a woman of great dignity and no matter how she felt, she was dressed in clean clothes, hair combed, and as always, there was the dangle of her gold charm bracelet on her arm. She was a lady to the end. She was still on her feet three days before she died, held upright by dignity alone. She loved politics and practically until her last breath was expressing her concern for the country.

She was a role model for me to watch as she faced her pain. She steadily slipped in height, but she grew in stature. Unknown to her, she had her own mission. Her courage was well known and her spunk, enthusiasm and intelligence were admired by many.

Her faith was strong. She was without fear as I watched her day by day. Though she would never have used his services, she would have her days where she would laugh through her pain and say, "Where's Dr. Kevorkian when you need him?"

She made me laugh too. Once again, the family's weird sense of humor came into play.

She died the most glorious death. My last view of her was in her own living room, in the hospice bed, with her dog nearby. As I peeked in, she had her hands raised to the ceiling She was gesturing and talking to my deceased father, by name, in the strong voice that might have belonged to a thirty year old. I watched and listened. Her facts and thoughts were absolutely clear. She was telling him details of my evening out. She did not know I was there.

As she finished and laid her hands on her chest, she could not speak to me. The hospice nurse told me she was in transition, no longer able to communicate with me, but communicating with those she saw before her. It was joyous. It was a supreme gift to me from her. My faith grew by bounds. I had not been near death before, but watching peace envelop her will always be the greatest gift she could have given me.

I have taken inventory of my life. I have counted my blessings. Born into a loving home to caring parents, I was never in want. I've had life-long friends. I have had education and travel. My devoted husband of 42 years is the joy of my life. We have raised two wonderful sons and now have been blessed by an incredible, loving daughter-in-law. I have lived to hold my beautiful grandchildren. If my life ended tomorrow, I could only be grateful for what God has given to me.

There is not a day in my life that I do not think of melanoma. My prognosis is encouraging, but melanoma will always be hanging over my head. My choice is to just, "Let go and let God." I am in His hands. I claim His promises.

"Yea though I walk through the valley of the shadow of death, I fear no evil, for Thou art with me." It says so in the Good Book.

Cancer isn't all bad. It's an opportunity to find out what is really important and grab it with gusto.

CHAPTER 10 - MY MISSION

Can anything good come of a possibly fatal disease? While I never ask, "Why Me?", I did ask, "How can this terrible thing be used for good?"

Every person reacts to this his or her own way. What works for one does not work for another. I knew that somehow I needed to gather my thoughts, my strengths, my capabilities, my skills, and use them to fight not only for myself, but for my family and others. I had no idea what path I would take. I just knew that I had to make lemonade out of this lemon I had been given.

Just getting the news and processing it is different for each individual. Some want to broadcast it. Some do not want anyone to know, want no sympathy, don't want to talk about it. Some want to walk the road alone, almost as if it is an embarrassment to have the disease.

You can figure out pretty quickly the type I am. After telling my family, I was quickly on the phone to my close friends, eliciting their support. My circle was wide, but I did not reach out to distant acquaintances. Perhaps I was one of those who was embarrassed to have the disease. I have a rather strong personality and somehow felt weakened by this pronouncement that I had encountered something I was not strong enough to defeat. Perhaps it was my ego that was damaged as much as my cells.

My decision to keep my condition somewhat confined was taken out of my hands. Every year I attend a charity brunch which supports cancer treatment at our local Hoag Memorial Hospital. It is attended by around 700 people, mostly women, many of whom I have known for years. Most of them had no idea I had had any problems at all.

Just a couple of months after my diagnosis, it was time for the brunch. The speaker asked all cancer survivors to stand. It took me by surprise. I froze. My mind raced into panic mode.

To stand up would be to admit my melanoma problem to the world. To stand up would tell them I was now in a weakened condition. There is that ego I was talking about. I did not want to be viewed as imperfect or weak. Not to stand was more of a problem. It was dishonest. I was a cancer survivor, even if at that point I had only survived two months.

It was an emotional moment for me as I slowly rose. I felt so obvious standing. I didn't belong with that group. I could see others for whom I had prayed, others who had lost their hair and were wearing wigs, others who had been damaged, but I also saw many who stood tall and strong. They were proud to be standing, proud to be alive. It was a moment of truth for me. It was like the feeling of the jarring cold that hits when one first dives into the ocean. I had joined them and had let the world know that, "I was one of them."

As I sat down I felt as if I had totally exposed myself. I had made the statement. I began to feel glad it was finally out in the open.

After the brunch, several confronted me. "What has happened?" "Where is it?" "Oh I am so sorry. I will pray for you."

Rather than feeling as if I had been reduced in people's minds, I found that their kindness and concern buoyed me and encouraged me. They cared more than I realized. The next year, I found myself ready to stand again. I thought, "Wow, I have made it another year. I am a cancer survivor."

In the market, people I barely knew would approach me and tell me they were praying for me. What had I done to deserve their concern?

I found myself fielding many questions about melanoma. It became common for people to show me their spots and to want my opinion. "Did your melanoma look like this?" I would direct them to their doctors.

I was very concerned that I was becoming a cocktail party bore. Sometimes it seemed as if people wanted to discuss melanoma. Other times I felt as if they wanted to escape from me. I made them nervous. It was very hard to draw the line between answering questions and not scaring people.

When people saw me with my head scarf on, they were reminded that the scarf was there because it covered the scar from a melanoma. They realized that their dermatologist had never checked their scalp, or they had had a bump on their head they should have checked. They went home vowing to make an appointment the next day.

I could feel myself being drawn into a mission of building melanoma awareness. It was time for melanoma to come out of the closet.

I wrote a paper , "Things You Need to Know about Melanoma." My oncologist checked it for accuracy. First it went to my Christmas card list. People told me they had mailed it to their Christmas card lists. I was being taken seriously.

The next copies of my papers went to the pastors of my church, since they deal with illness so much. They would encounter melanoma patients at times.

My phone began to ring. "Would you talk to my friend?" "Would you call my brother?" Calls came from Colorado, Hawaii, Indiana, Washington. I found out that I could calm people. I could help them prepare questions to ask of their doctors. If the call came before the biopsy, I could educate them about the punch biopsy and the Sentinel Node procedure. Several actually made appointments with my oncologist, Dr. Bilchik, at John Wayne Cancer Institute.

I wrote a second paper to clarify some of the things from my first paper. My papers have been circulated to thousands. They are on the internet at **www.themelanomaletter.com**. Many have taken them to their skin doctors. Some skin doctors are interested. Some are not.

People continued to ask me about melanoma. They wanted to know how it was found, what it looked like and the treatment I was receiving. In a sermon, our pastor spoke of each of us finding our own ministry. It seemed as if I had a ministry calling I would never have expected.

My papers have apparently helped to build awareness and promote prevention. My mission began to take shape. For years volunteering in the community was part of my schedule. I had held responsible positions in my church. My original occupation had been teaching school. My whole adult life was spent being a wife and mother. I had run a business. All of these things were beginning to meld together.

Meetings were no longer simple to attend. When I scheduled things I often had to cancel for some health appointment. That pressure was not needed in my life.

My mission was right in front of me, my telephone, and my

computer. I could sit at my desk and communicate with others by phone and e-mail.

Thus it has gone. There is barely a week that goes by without a call from someone. Just having someone neutral to talk to is all the help that is needed. I am an anonymous person. Most of my melanoma friends I never meet face to face. I am there to walk through the crisis with them. Once they are into their treatment of choice, we often drift apart. I will get an occasional update.

Sometimes the phone doesn't ring again. I was very concerned about one man I had talked with many times, though had never met. He came to me in a rather unusual way.

Two friends were at a restaurant one evening about nine o'clock. As they started to leave, the solo man at the next booth stopped them. He told them he had heard them talking about cancer and that he had melanoma and was so scared. They offered to have me call him and at ten that night we connected.

He was so frightened. He knew he was probably facing death and he had no one to talk to. My emphasis was in talking to those who were living with melanoma. I wasn't quite sure how to handle talking with someone who might lose the battle. I sensed he was not a person of faith. We talked for quite a while and I tried to comfort him. I called him a couple of other times and he was trying new treatments. Then I called and his phone had been disconnected. No forwarding number. I regret that I did not pray with him. He might not have rejected my prayer. It might have comforted him. I pray he has found his peace.

I knew he was pursuing some treatment in Switzerland at one time. Wouldn't it be wonderful if I received a call from him that his phone was disconnected because he was in Switzerland....LIVING. It could be!!

I had talked death with my mother as she faced her mortality at 89. She taught me so much. I remember the day I had to call her and say her cancer had returned after five years. She replied, "Well, I am just not going to worry about it. Would you stop and get me a Kentucky Fried Chicken dinner ?" I was fascinated. I will never forget it. She knew what my pronouncement meant. She had already decided there would be no more treatment. My mother had her bags packed and faced death head on. But for the time being, she would just go on living, Thank You!

She was a person of deep faith. She had no worries about her soul. The natural ebb of life and death became so apparent to me. The realization that every person we know will walk the path someday, each one of us in a different way, but we will all walk the path. We are all terminal. We just don't know when.

I know that melanoma has its eye on its victims. None of us know which ones it will take. All of us need help in facing the facts, in walking the road. We need to be here for each other and to see the beauty of each day as we live it. I hope I can keep my perspective and help others. Helping others is a great gift to me.

Each new day of my mission brings a new situation. Sometimes I will be put in touch with the patient at the very beginning. I feel really good when that happens. I can explain melanoma, give them questions to ask, suggest getting second opinions, teach them about punch biopsies and the Sentinel Node procedure.

I am very careful to remind them that they are talking to a lay person, just another traveler on the road. I have no medical skills.

I am just a teaching tool.

My friend living in the northwest had a suspicious but rather unremarkable spot under her tongue. It could have been something as simple as a freckle, perhaps an amalgam tattoo from a filling or.....possibly, a melanoma. It was a difficult call for her doctors in the north. Knowing it had a minute chance of being malignant, they really didn't want to surgically remove it without a diagnosis. If it was removed, they would have possibly wrecked her chance for the Sentinel Node test, which they did not have the facilities to do. Because of my paper, she ultimately flew to California to have it removed by my oncologist. Since she had had a melanoma in her past, it had to be considered that this could be one too.

Dr. Bilchik had to proceed with the surgery in the knowledge that she might need to have the Sentinel Node surgery done on the spot. He sent her to have the Sentinel Node mapping as a precaution, and had a pathologist ready in the operating room, for an immediate diagnosis. It was benign, thank goodness, and he did not have to continue with the Sentinel Node test. Dr. Bilchik could just remove the spot, which turned out to be amalgam , and sew her up. At her follow up exam, he told her that he had seen melanoma on the tongue before, so her trip had not been wasted. It was the right thing to do.

The exciting thing for me is that my mission has spawned its first missionary. She is very happy with what she has learned about melanoma, and her doctors who did not know about the Sentinel Node procedure will soon know what it is all about. She went home armed with informational papers from the John Wayne Cancer Institute.

One of her doctors was not pleased when she asked for a punch biopsy. In fact he was very resistant, telling her he had removed melanomas for thirty years by just scooping them out. She resisted and told him what she knew from my paper. She saw him later and he said, "Did you say the person who wrote the paper (meaning me) was still alive?" She told him I was. He replied, "Amazing!!" Apparently she got him to do a little further thinking on the matter.

A doctor teaching in one of the medical schools near my friend sent his students home to research the the Sentinel Node procedure on the internet and report on it. The next class of graduates will know. My student has become very knowledgeable about melanoma. She has made me proud.

My mission has given purpose to my melanoma. I am so thrilled to have a part in possibly saving someone else's life. It has brought me great joy. I thank God for giving me something of value to teach others. It is a privilege to be put in touch with people who just need a hand to hold.

CHAPTER 11 - YOUR MISSION

You can help too, you know. There is plenty of work for all of us.

Since we have a good idea that sun could be a big factor in this, the first job is sun protection for you, your family, and your friends.

Let's start with sun lotion. It doesn't do any good in the bottle. Carry it with you and slather it on all over yourself. If you are thin on top, don't forget the top of your head is closer to the sun than the rest of you. Do it on those days where it doesn't seem sunny, because those rays are coming through.

It is critically important to get your kids to stand still for a few moments of slathering. Many times I have watched mothers put lotion all over baby's skin and face and ignore the baby fine hair on top the head. Go on and rub it in. It will wash out soon enough. Do it several times a day.

Pick your time for sunning. Those midday hours are the killers. My husband and I spend a lot of time on the beach, but we are under a leafy spreading tree. We have the enjoyment of the beach, with the effects of the rays considerably minimized. Of course we have our lotion on and usually our hats.

Beach umbrellas are better than nothing, but many are really too thin to do the job well. You can still see shadows on the beach towel. Sun is getting through. Don't just leave baby sleeping under one and think he is protected. I have actually found a beach umbrella that advertises 35 SPF and I will sometimes put it up, under the tree, for extra protection.

Finally, analyzing that visors were a culprit for my problem, I am always in a hat. If you can get one on your child you will be doing him or her a favor. Wearing one yourself sets a good example.

There are many lines of clothing that have sun protection. My favorite is Sun Precautions, sold by catalog.(1-800-882-7860). I always put it on for swimming or boating. This clothing is actually designated by the F.D.A.as "a medical device." It comes in many colors and styles for golfers, hikers, swimmers, and just everyday life. There are lots of things for children. It was developed by a man who had had his own bout with melanoma and decided to do something to help others.

Don't fool yourself that putting a t-shirt on is helping much. A tee might only give you 7 or 8 SPF protection and less than that if it gets wet.

One bad sunburn in your youth could eventually be the area where skin cancer might attack. Teach your children why covering up is important.

We all admire the healthy, robust, look of a suntanned beach goer. It really does look great unless it has reached the leathery look. I used to adore being tan. In fact, I must admit, I was somewhat proud of my tan. I not only baked in it, I added plenty of baby oil to make sure I fried. I really didn't burn, however, just a nice color. Well, look at me now, fighting for my life because of those decisions I made long years ago. We didn't have the knowledge then that we do now. Learn about it and take it seriously.

Talk to your tennis buddies and your golf partners. In the years of my problems, so many of my friends have told me that they have started wearing hats. They never analyzed visors. Like many of you, I didn't want to mess up my hair with a hat. A visor had a sportier look. Well, I am paying the price. I cringe when I see the noonday tennis courts full of visor clad players.

If I have a friend who has something unusual looking on the skin, I bring it up. Perhaps they know nothing of melanoma. You don't have to be scary, just a little suggestion that they should have a dermatologist check them out will do. Some people I have met have never even seen a dermatologist.

Support melanoma research. Make others aware of the need. Volunteer your services. Attend fund raising functions. Those of us under treatment have been the beneficiaries of time, money and effort by throngs of other people. It is payback time. We need to show our appreciation by doing our part.

Express appreciation to those who are part of your treatment. They need a pat on the back just like everybody else.

Most of all, help spread the word about the Sentinel Node test. Spread it about melanoma and breast cancer. You don't have to go into detail. Just make your friends aware enough to see if their doctors use those techniques. Somewhere, someone's life could be saved.

CHAPTER 12 - TIPS FOR TREATMENT

Along the way I have done a few things that have made my walk easier. By far the best one done is a computer printout of my entire health history.

It begins with my broken nose at six years old and follows through my entire memory of things which might have had some lasting effects such as unexplained scars, inoculations, tetanus shots, whatever I could think of.

Each new doctor's office or test I have, I am presented with pages to fill out. I answer the questions I can and then just say, "See attached." It has made my life so much easier. Can you imagine trying to explain nine surgeries on two lines?

Included on my sheets are all of my medications, complete with dosage. I have listed my various scans, colonoscopies, and x-rays chronologically, along with a short statement such as , "Clear" or "All OK."

My insurance information and phone numbers for my family are on it.

Finally I have listed my family history and the names, specialty, phone and FAX numbers of all my doctors. I update the list on the computer with each event and make sure that I have a copy with me at all times. It takes much of the exasperation out of filling out more forms.

When I have tests that are yearly or important enough that a new doctor might be interested in them, I will often ask for a copy for my files. I do this more with lab tests than anything, so I can keep a small record for myself. I have copies of most of my tests sent to my internist also.

Sometimes things can be made easier by just asking your doctor for other ways to do them. Every month I had to take special blood tests a week after my vaccine. That would have meant an extra trip to Santa Monica each month. My doctor gave me the proper test tubes and orders and I went in to my local hospital in Newport Beach, Hoag Memorial Hospital, Presbyterian, for the blood test on the correct day. They would pack my serum in ice and I would take it home and freeze it until I was due for another vaccine treatment. It was great.

Many of my scans and tests were taken in my local area too. The only negative is that it takes a little longer for the results to reach the doctor, so more waiting.

Speaking of scans or MRI's, do they bother you? I am a bit claustrophobic so I do not look forward to them. My secret is to close my eyes before they roll me into any tube. I never open my eyes inside the tube. If I did I would get real antsy. Keeping them closed and trying some of my sleep memory work, I have never had a problem with them.

It is very important to make sure that whatever medical product you are ingesting does not interfere with something else you are taking. For instance, it was very important for me to know that taking cortisone could possibly nullify the positive effects of the vaccine I was taking. I am very careful to run any new medications or changes by my oncologist.

I was taking a strong herbal remedy to help my immune system once, and when I began a new medication on top of the herbs there was a reaction. I stopped the herbs immediately. Even though they are natural, the combination can have a strong effect.

There are days when I would just love a massage. There are conflicting views on whether massage is good for cancer patients. Some in that field feel that the last thing a cancer patient should do is try to move cells around the body. Others report finding no negative effects from the results of their studies. I think you should discuss it with your oncologist and make up your own mind. My oncologist did not seem concerned when I ask him about it, but I have been a little nervous about doing it.

Make a note to remember to see your regular doctors for checkups. When dealing with cancer it is easy to concentrate on that and forget things like colonoscopies, or other yearly routine tests for cholesterol and heart.

Lastly, I have been fortunate that my husband has driven me to all my vaccine appointments. Most of the time he is in the waiting room. On "Decision Days" I think it is critical to have another set of ears in the room. Sometimes there is more than one way to handle something and it needs to be analyzed. Other times, there is just a lot of information dispelled, and it is very helpful to have someone else hear it.

All of this falls into a routine along the way. As you keep reappearing at various check-in desks, it all becomes familiar. You have an extended family who will be glad to see you. I always feel happy to step off the elevator and see Rob or Beth, the receptionists, smiling at me. By the time I get to the lab, Merry Larry, the Happy Vampire, is ready to entertain me while drawing my blood. My nurse, Lynn, and I hug and catch up. Maryellen and Maria, Mary, Heather, and Joan, are usually rushing from duty to duty. I swap stories with Dr. Bilchik. They are my team. They are a rich part of my life. I am so grateful for them.

CHAPTER 13 - THE FAMILY FACTOR

Cancer is a family disease. When it hits one, it hits all, It is not easy to ignore. There are appointments, tests, surgeries, emotions, decisions and always the apprehensive waiting for results.

The fine line that must be drawn is between talking about your situation enough to be able to cope with it and not becoming so consumed that no one wants to hear another word.

In my case, my husband has been on the front lines with me every step of the way. He has never uttered a complaint, and more than that has told me he was happy to be there for me and wouldn't have it any other way. This devotion is a gift from God, and I know that not all who are facing these kinds of decisions and traumas are as fortunate as I have been. I know I am blessed. I hope you have someone close to you who will walk this path with you, discuss your fears and decisions.

If you are that companion, thank you. You are so important to your loved one. Your willingness to walk this walk is the greatest gift one might give another.

Every member of the family will handle it in a different way. Our family relies on humor. I suppose someone hearing us might think we are an insensitive bunch, but we know what we mean and don't mean. When my son says to me, "Mom, when you die, can I have the gold in your teeth?" I just laugh-Hey, if he wants to go after it, he can have it. I have seen the looks on faces, when he says something like that to me, and I can't believe how shocked some people can be. I guess we are just weird.

When God created me, I know He mistakenly gave me an extra set of worry genes. Knowing that, He gave me sons to make sure those genes would be used.

I have coped with broken bones, car crashes, driving 110 miles per hour, girlfriends, skiing black diamond runs, sailing oceans on small boats, and even a plane crash. Now I find out there were things I didn't even know about and I should have been using those genes more.

I don't think I have given my sons much to worry about until now. We don't talk about it a lot. I keep them posted on major issues. but I try to keep the minor stuff out of the picture. Their dad and I are handling it. I do know, however, that if there is a need, they will be there for me. How do I know? Because I saw them with their grandmother. The morning after she was diagnosed they were at her hospital bedside helping her to make decisions. They became totally involved in encouraging her to fight. They kept track of her by phone and visits. They ran errands. They showed their care in many ways. I know from what I saw then that they would be at my side in a minute. Of course, when they read this they will probably have some great wisecracks, but I know them too well.

My daughter-in-law is one for whom family is all important. I know that she too would be there for me. She still wonders at the wisecracks, however. That wouldn't be her way, but she would bring a caring strength and willingness if she was needed.

Our grandchildren would continue to provide the joy that only they can muster.

Knowing that they would be there if needed, I would rather spend my time with them just enjoying their positive humor. I am excited about what they are doing in their lives, and I would much rather talk about that. I am excited to be with our grandchildren and feel so grateful that we all live close.

Because of the hereditary nature of some cancers, it is important to be totally honest about diagnosis and treatment. Hopefully your family will not need the information, but it should be in their memory log. It should be something they are aware of for their children.

My advice is to waste very little time discussing your woes with your family. Families are to be enjoyed and loved, not burdened unless necessary.

CHAPTER 14 - THE COCKTAIL PARTY

Have you ever been trapped at a party by someone anxious to share their aches and pains with you? You glance at others who are laughing and telling stories. How you wish you could escape.

It usually starts with an inquiry about your health, and quickly deteriorates to, "Let me tell you about mine."

I have to entertain the real possibility that I may be a total bore to some people. Boy, it is hard to even think that, but I know there is truth to it. I can feel it happening at times, and I get in so deep that I can't backtrack gracefully. I am even boring myself.

As much as I try to downplay my problems, one person can innocently inquire about my health, and then mention that they know someone newly diagnosed, and it sets me off. I have to know all the details. Maybe I have a mission here. I am sure there are people who wish they had never asked in the first place.

People care, but they really don't want to be bogged down with your problems. They have enough of their own. Besides, they came to a party.

I think the hardest thing to do is to be truthful and yet not lay your worries on someone else. I spend a lot of my life waiting for ominous tests. Biopsies and tests can take as much as ten days. Something suspicious has been detected. There is an ominous possibility and it must be looked at. The tests are done. The wait is on. About then, a cocktail party has shown up on the calendar.

"How are you doing?" Pause. I think, "I wonder how I am doing.

I wonder if the test will be good or bad. What is my answer to this simple question?" How AM I doing? I finally learned to say, "Today is Great!"

Among close friends, I might say, "Well I am waiting for some more results." Then I ask myself why I burdened them with that. Why should I give my dear friends cause to worry. That is rather sadistic of me to do. I am doing enough worrying for everybody. I have tried to come up with, "As far as I know everything is great." That is the truth. At that moment in time, I don't know anything else. That is an answer that satisfies people, and I can go back to my own worries.

One thing I resort to at times is to have something in mind before a deep conversation begins. I love books. A good book or a new movie is always fodder for turning the conversation. It can head the melanoma drama off at the pass. I don't even care for baseball, but "How 'bout those Angels?" "I hear you spent three months in Provence." We are off and running now.

If you are having problems like this, give it a little thought before you hit the party. It is a skill you need to acquire. I work on it all the time.

It is very easy to become a one issue person. There is so much going on in this world. You know it is a strange thing. You and I have had our health threatened, but at this moment in time the whole world is threatened. Nations have the capabilities to create the great Armageddon. We are not the only ones living in fear. The world is. It is just a different kind of fear.

Again, you don't need to worry about that too. Our leaders have taken on that responsibility. Release that worry to them.

In fact, confine your worries to those things you can do something about. One of those things is your health and your treatment. This is your time to concentrate on you. This is your time to push away those extra things that upset you. I will try to do the same thing, too.

Let's arm ourselves for that cocktail party and pick the funniest guy there to talk to. Let's plan to come home laughing.

CHAPTER 15 - THE NEW PERSPECTIVE

Have you noticed that mirrors change as you age? Those bright eyes, that smooth skin, that hourglass figure or those bulging biceps all seem to let Mother Nature have her way. We see the blooms on flowers wilt, the leaves change colors and fall. It is all so natural, unless it happens to us, and then we fight it with all we have.

My community probably has more plastic surgeons than it has regular doctors. It is full of beautiful people who work out at gyms and keep themselves beautiful. It is a challenge to the rest of us.

Social gatherings often reduce to analyzing the latest diet craze. People disappear and emerge with new faces, new shapes. Makeup is perfect. Clothes are stylish. It isn't hard to envy perfection.

As I have aged, the scales have not been good to me. My youthful energy has succumbed to bad knees and the pull of gravity. I hide the fact that my naturally blond hair has had some occasional help. People have always admired my smooth tan. I used to be proud of it. How mixed up can priorities get!

When disease hits the body, it hits the body image too. All of a sudden, the spare tire doesn't seem so important. Comfort food takes on new importance for some. It isn't the right way to handle a crisis, but it does give a temporary good feeling. Others don't want to eat a thing and lose weight. Neither way is good.

Health far outweighs beauty, but it is hard to concentrate on outward health when inner health is suffering.

In my case, I began to ignore my extra pounds. When a woman

has two large permanent bald spots on the front of her head, it becomes more of a focus than the weight. Those secrets that only my hairdresser knows were put on the back burner. After my surgeries, I really didn't want anyone messing around with my hair.

Stress brings out a few new lines and wrinkles that don't seem to want to go away. I found myself not really caring. On a good day I put on lipstick, but the eyeliner became a chore I didn't need.

Slowly, a new perspective began to grow within me. The realization that life isn't a competition grew. The inner self became the only really important bloom and if it would grow and bloom, the outer self would reflect that growth. We all remember when we were young and felt ugly and our mothers used to say, "Just wait." They had already learned that inner beauty is what is important. We probably didn't believe our mothers, but you know, they were right.

It is not how you look to others that counts. It is how you look to yourself.

As I have gradually gotten a handle on this I have taken a few steps forward. I have tried to build a Happy Face from within. While driving I have become conscious of the vacant negative stare I might have on my face. I turn it into a smile. There is some saying about how many fewer muscles it takes to smile than to frown. It really does change the atmosphere in the car. The red light is no longer so annoying.

A little eyeliner really does make me perk up. I don't care if anybody else notices. I notice and I feel better.

The pounds annoy me, but I limit myself to climbing one mountain at a time. Maybe when I reach the crest of this mountain I will make another stab at the weight mountain, but for now it will have to wait. For now, I will concentrate on the mountain of wellness.

The true realization is that the people who are dearest to me have ridden up and down the scale with me. Those who judge me by my hair style, my makeup or my weight are not the life companions who mean the most to me. Those who cherish what I am within are the ones I hold most dear.

A plastic surgeon could send his kids to college on me, but it isn't going to happen. I agree with people who say, "I worked too hard to get these wrinkles, I'm not giving them up now." My world revolves around truth. What you see is what you get. My bald spots are here to stay.

What's really important? FAITH, LOVE, FAMILY, FRIENDSHIP, BLUE SKY, SMILES, TRUTH, GOODNESS, KINDNESS, LAUGHTER, PEACE, HEALTH, WORK, PLAY, HUGS,.....

What isn't important? Any disfiguring melanoma scar.

YOU ARE A MELANOMA PATIENT BUT...

You are an individual.

You are different from anyone else.

You are more than a statistic.

You may be in a program that is not represented in a statistical study.

You may have friends and family who pray for you regularly.

You have it within you to refuse to be a victim.

You are fighting back.

You may have an inner attitude that will not accept any negative thoughts.

You may be a miracle in the making.

You Remember That!!!

Now, let's get on with it and make Lemonade!!!

FELLOW "CLUB MELANOMA" MATES AND FRIENDS:

If you have gained any benefit from reading this material, please consider making a donation to assist in research to find a cure for melanoma.

Contributions will be welcomed by:

John Wayne Cancer Institute
"Lemons Make Lemonade Fund"
2001 Santa Monica Blvd, Suite 860-W
Santa Monica, CA 90404 USA

Hoag Hospital Foundation
"Lemons Make Lemonade Fund"
P.O. Box 6100
Newport Beach, CA 92663

Help to promote awareness, screenings, and community melanoma education by a contribution to:

Eisenhower Lucy Curci Cancer Center
Patient and Family Support Fund - "Lemonade"
39000 Bob Hope Drive
Rancho Mirage, CA 92270

JOIN THIS EFFORT TO HELP DEFEAT MELANOMA!
THANK YOU,

SALLY WELSH

An update of my cancer vaccine from the office of Dr. Donald L. Morton, Medical Director and Surgeon-in-Chief, The John Wayne Cancer Institute.

Late in the fall of 2005, the Data Safety Monitoring Committee recommended that the Canvaxin (melanoma vaccine) trial be discontinued. This was done because the third interim analysis found the data are unlikely to provide significant evidence of overall survival benefit for patients with stage III melanoma who were treated with Canvaxin plus BCG versus those who received placebo plus BCG. Because there are so few effective therapeutic options for this dreaded disease, this news was particularly disappointing.

However, there is some good news. The results of the trial set a new high standard for survival of stage III and stage IV melanoma. The other good news is that important information about the immunologic response to melanoma, molecular markers and diagnostic biomarkers were derived from the trial data. Important information regarding the biology of metastatic melanoma and the patient's immunologic response to the disease should be forthcoming. In the coming months the physicians and scientists will be working hard to pull and analyze the data to figure out what can be done to improve our vaccine. Based upon the results of these laboratory studies, a new vaccine will be developed by Dr. Morton and tested at the John Wayne Cancer Institute.

Surgical oncologists are still seeing melanoma patients at the John Wayne Cancer Institute which is currently one of the largest melanoma facilities in the world.